From Nurse to Educator:

Creating Effective Learning Experiences for Adults

by Lyla Berry, EdD, MA, RN

Credits

MANAGING EDITOR
Susan Alvare

COPY EDITOR
Susan Clair

COVER DESIGN
Kirsten Browne

INTERIOR DESIGN/COMPOSITION
Thaddeus Castillo/Susan Alvare

ILLUSTRATOR
Thaddeus Castillo

Copyright Information

Hartman Publishing, Inc.
8529-A Indian School Road NE
Albuquerque, NM 87112
(505) 291-1274
web: www.**hartman**online.com
e-mail: orders@hartmanonline.com

ISBN 1-888343-55-9

Acknowledgments

The publisher gratefully acknowledges the contributions of the following individuals who reviewed this material:

Betty Fay, RN, SDC, ICN
Genevieve Gipson, RN, MEd, RNC
Judith C. Goodwin, MSN, RN, CS, GNP
Katherine Purgatorio Howard, MSN, RNC
Leah Klusch, RN, BSN, MA
Catherine R. Van Son, RN, MSN
Katherine Vaughn, RN, BSN
Karen Walborn, PhD, RNCS
Judith A. Walker, PhD, RN

Excerpts from *Teach! Plain Talk About Teaching* by Leo A. Meyer, LAMA Books, Leo A. Meyer Associates, Hayward, CA reprinted by permission of the author.

From the author:

There are too many people who directly or indirectly contributed to this text to express my appreciation to them individually, including all of my past students. I wish to thank my parents for teaching me the invaluable lessons of caring and commitment. And my sincere appreciation to my daughter, T. Lynn Berry, an instructor herself, who suggestions and editing assistance were priceless.

Notice to the Reader

Table of Contents

Introduction

Teaching is an integral part of the nursing practice. Nursing professionals are involved on a daily basis teaching patient/client/residents, peers, or employees in a variety of healthcare settings.

I, like most nurses, arrived at my first nursing education position equipped only with experience and competent clinical skills. I thought teaching was telling.

I soon realized that the teaching profession and the nursing profession each possess a unique set of skills. The myth that "all nurses are teachers" is as absurd as stating that "all teachers are nurses." Nursing professionals involved with teaching need to be provided with information concerning adult teaching and learning principles, as well as how to utilize and incorporate those principles in planning, implementing, and presenting effective adult-learning experiences.

Teaching involves *context* as well as *content*. This concept may be illustrated by a simple comparison in which teaching is likened to a cup of coffee. The coffee is the *content*. The content is the information to be presented. The cup is the *context*. Teaching without the context is like giving someone coffee without the cup. The *context provider* is the instructor, who gives the content structure, purpose, and meaning.

This is the wonderful challenge of teaching, trying

to meet the needs of each student, as in nursing one strives to meet the needs of each patient/client/resident.

This text was specifically developed to assist the licensed nursing professional directly involved in the role of adult teaching in all healthcare facility or nursing school setting.

Happy Teaching!

1 What is Adult Learning?

Learning has been described in various texts as a product, process, or function in which transformation occurs, leading to an internal process. This internal process, in turn, leads to a behavioral change through the altering of one's insights, problem-solving techniques, expectations, and/or thought patterns.

Learning is not simply the acquisition of knowledge, but it is the ability to *apply* that knowledge through the use of appropriate judgment and decision making. Learning is the changing of thoughts, ideas or attitudes, and behavior.

Learning has been defined as:
- a product: the acquisition and mastery of that which one already knows; an outcome of an experience.
- a process: the organized, intentional testing of ideas relevant to problems and a mechanism by which behavior is changed, shaped, or controlled.
- a function: an extension and clarification of the meanings of one's experience; a change that can motivate acquiring new information based on connections that relate to both the new and familiar.

To live is to learn. Learning continues throughout life whether intentional or unintentional, formal or informal. Much is learned through the socialization process from family upbringing, peer influences, and the media. Learning pertains to life experiences, both positive and negative. Learning can take place by example. Consider these facts about learning:

- Learning is an everyday process, from academic programs to learning how to use a new appliance. However, learning is not always the result of a deliberate effort.
- Learning can be intuitive. Knowledge can come from within by creative insights and thoughts.
- Learning is congruent with human development. Learning affects and is affected by the biological and physical changes in personality, values, roles, and tasks that occur over a normal span of life.
- Children learn differently from adults. Adults have experienced more than children, and those experiences represent a rich resource. Even so, they may be obstacles to learning because adult learning includes, in part, a process of reaffirming, recognizing, and reintegrating one's previous experience, which is not the case with children. Adults have developed a more-delayed gratification process. Children are dependent, adults are (or should be) independent.
- Learning is a personal and natural process. Learning takes place within the person, and this process continues to evolve from birth.
- Learning can be enhanced by those who take per-

sonal responsibility for learning and through self-motivation.

- Learning involves change. Change may produce anxiety and resistance or fear of the unknown. Adults seek learning experiences, at times, to cope with specific life-changing events.

There are two common misunderstandings that exist that are associated with teaching adults. One is the belief that when all the facts and information have been presented, learning takes place.

Teaching isn't telling. The fact that information is presented is no guarantee that learning took place. The mere reciting of information does not guarantee understanding of the information. Although the presenting of knowledge is an important function of education, the educator must ascertain the degree of understanding.

Example:

> First little girl: "I taught my dog, Spot, to whistle."
>
> Second little girl: "I don't hear him whistling."
>
> First little girl: "I said I taught him. I didn't say he learned it."

The second misunderstanding is the belief that all learning takes place in the classroom.

Learning does not always occur in the classroom. Learning pertains to experience or experiencing. Learning experiences can occur in any place or at any time. Probably one of the most important methods of teaching is by example. People learn from watching and listening to others. Learning can be achieved by doing and observing, and learning can, as, previously stated, can also be intuitive.

The desired result of learning is a change in behavior, which may involve mental, emotional, or physical activity. Learning is the change in thoughts, ideas, or attitudes.

What are the basic principles of learning?

Learning encompasses many concepts. Here are a few important points to know:

- Learning is an experience that occurs within the learner and is activated by the learner. The learner mostly controls the process of learning. Teaching is facilitating. Learners learn what they *want* to learn; there must be personal involvement on the part of the learner.
- Learning is the discovery of personal meaning and relevance of ideas. The learner is more likely to internalize the concepts and ideas relevant to his/her needs and problems.
- Learning is a consequence of experience. For example, people become responsible not from having been told to be responsible, but from having experienced responsibility.
- Learning is a collaborative process. Interaction helps validate one's sense of identity and gain confidence in giving, sharing, and learning together. The interactive aspect of learning encourages creativity.

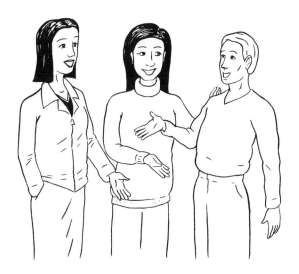

• Learning is an evolutionary process. For lasting learning, time and patience are required. Adults learn better in an atmosphere that fosters active and personal involvement, allows free and open communication, acceptance (the right to make mistakes), and respect.

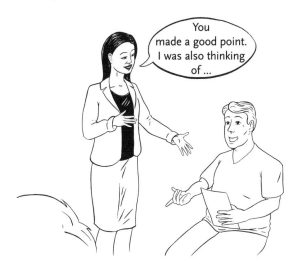

- Learning is sometimes a painful process. Often, behavioral change involves giving up that which is comfortable for new ways of doing or thinking.
- One of the richest resources for learning is the learner.
- The learner brings an accumulation of experiences, ideas, feelings, and attitudes to the learning process.

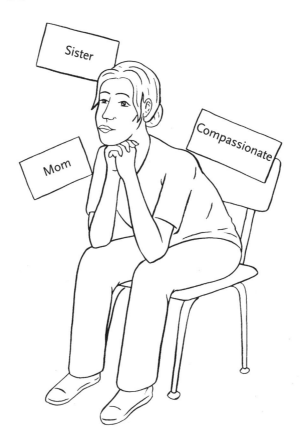

- The process of learning is emotional as well as intellectual.
- Learning is enhanced when a person's feelings and thoughts are in harmony.
- Behavior that is rewarded is more likely to recur.

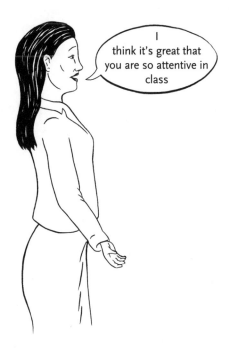

- Compliment learners evenly. It is easy to compliment a good student, but the educator must try harder to encourage the slower learner. Remember: almost everyone does at least one thing well.
- Classroom/group atmosphere affects satisfaction in learning.

Knowles's Core Principles of Adult Learning

Adult learning theory is based on six major assumptions, which differentiate the education of adults from the education of children. Malcolm Knowles, one of the most referenced authorities on adult learning, describes new perspectives about teaching and elaborates on applying the core principles of adult learning:

1. The learner's need to know

Adults should have their need to learn recognized and have input into what, why, and how they will learn.

2. Self-concept of the learner

Adults should believe that what is learned bears meaning.

3. Prior experience of the learner

Prior experience can be a rich resource or create a bias that influences the shape of new learning. It can provide grounding for the adult's self-identity and create a wider range of individual differences.

4. Readiness to learn

The level or readiness of an adult is closely associated to the need to know. Readiness to learn can be encouraged by direction, support, and encouragement. Life's situations can also create a need to know.

5. Orientation to learning

Adults generally prefer a problem-solving orientation to learning, rather than a subject-centered
learning. Learning is created through transformation of experience. The individual's cognitive ability influences cognitive controls, which influence
cognitive styles, which, in turn, influence learning
styles.

6. Motivation to learn

Adults tend to be more motivated toward learning
that helps them solve problems in their lives or
results from internal or external payoffs. This can
be in the form of success, value, enjoyment, or a
sense of choice in the learning process.

What are basic guidelines for instruction?

From the core assumptions, the nurse educator
may identify some basic guidelines upon which to
direct instruction. All of the following statements
may not apply in every situation or for every learner. Some statements may be overlapping, and
some may seem to be contradictory. However, they
are worthy of consideration:

The adult learner:
- should experience success and encouragement
  frequently
- has past experiences and values that affect what
  he or she perceives
- responds to frequent changes in method

- must see relevance of class learning experiences to his or her own life and activities
- may be motivated by some force, such as certification, promotion, or a pay increase
- should be treated as an adult
- is more committed to an activity for which he or she has participated in the planning stages
- will have more success in a problem-centered curriculum
- may suffer more-frequent fatigue, which may be a negative factor in learning
- is more likely to have established habits
- may have external distractions, such as work, family, or money problems
- may be more sensitive to criticism

What are the best conditions for adult learning in a healthcare facility?

Healthcare management must regard employee training and development as a long-range process, requiring investment in time and effort. If healthcare facilities are to minimize employee turnover and maximize productivity, it is essential that those responsible for developing and training be aware of the employee's needs. Administrators cannot afford to have a casual attitude about training or be unaware of the serious problems that can result from poor instruction. Consider these conditions:

- The employee must first recognize some unfulfilled need and view his or her employment as contributing to the satisfaction of this need.

- The employee must consider the job to be a desirable means to fulfilling a goal and obtaining recognition.
- The employee must be motivated to become a productive worker. The organizational climate and the actions and behavior of the supervisor are important to creating motivation.
- The learning process must be directed toward providing the employee with acceptable levels of success and failure.
- The employee brings his or her prior job experiences, habits, and values to the learning experience. These factors affect attitudes and perceptions.
- The learning process must permit the integration of new job knowledge with that which the employee already knows.
- The employee will consider the performance of a new procedure as positive only if he or she understands why it is personally important.
- The employee must be given an opportunity to participate in developing changes and improvements in the job for which he or she is responsible.

What do adult learners bring to the classroom?

In addition to individual differences and student characteristics, the adult learner brings these more-significant resources to the classroom:

Motivation

Motivation is probably the most important condition for learning. If the student is not motivated to learn, learning will not take place. Motivation is an internal experience that is activated by the learner. Students learn what they choose to learn. There must be a personal involvement on the part of the learner.

Students may be in a classroom for various reasons, ranging from required attendance to having a desire to learn as much as they can. For some, motivation may be the result of job requirements; for others, to secure a better salary or for self-improvement. For most, motivation levels fall somewhere between those who are willing to be in class and those who are totally unwilling to be in class. Most students in job-related classes can understand and appreciate the connection between what they learn and what they earn.

Although teaching is facilitating, an instructor can influence motivation by creating a need to learn. When a need has been established, some form of behavior change will be displayed. An individual with high self-esteem will tend to be motivated to perform well in class. However, a teacher can assist in building a stronger sense of self-esteem for students by giving them confidence that they can master the skills and knowledge they are studying. Wlodowski (1985) suggests a model of characteristics and skills for instructors to apply to be good motivators of adults.

Characteristics and skills of motivating instructors are grouped into four categories:

1. Expertise – knowledge and preparation skills necessary to convey information.

2. Empathy – understanding and consideration; a realistic understanding of the learner's needs and expectations, and the ability to adapt instruction to the level of the learner.

3. Enthusiasm – caring about and valuing that which is being taught; expressed commitment with appropriate degrees of emotion, animation, and energy.

4. Clarity – power of language and organization; can be understood and followed by most learners, and provides a way to comprehend what has been taught.

There are three primary components that act as motivators for adult learning: life changes, increasing self-esteem, and integrating new ideas into old ones.

Life changes influence adults in that they often seek learning experiences to cope with these events. They will also seek learning experiences that will enhance job advancement or build self-esteem. If they are going to use and keep the new information, adults need to be able to integrate new ideas with what they already know. Information that conflicts with what they hold to be true forces a reevaluation of the old material, and information is integrated more slowly.

Ability

The ability to learn is nearly as important as motivation. A student with limited ability but plenty of
motivation and determination will often out-per-
form the genius with a bad attitude. Although
motivation may be the most critical factor, ability
counts for a lot. Some students may be limited in
intellectual ability; this is a factor that the educator
has no control over and cannot change, but at least
the educator can attempt to motivate students to do
their best. Some students may be limited by a lack
of basic skills; however, this is *not* the same as lack-
ing the ability to learn.

Attitude

Students bring a mixture of diverse cultural, social,
and economic and backgrounds. Students also
bring with them various combinations of knowledge, abilities, and attitudes. In addition, they may
all have different reactions to the educator. Letting
students know that the educator's goal is to help
them to succeed will overcome a major hurdle.
Students sense whether the educator wants to be
in the classroom or is merely going through the
motions. Let students know that learning can be
fun, and that learning occurs best when students
learn together.

What are some differences among adult learners?

The major premise of research on individual differences is that instructors should adapt instruction

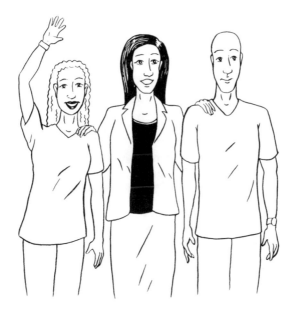

to accommodate differences in individual abilities, styles, and preferences. Individuals vary in their approaches, strategies, and preferences during learning activities. Jonassen and Grabowski (1993) describe three broad categories of individual differences that impact learning:

Cognitive Differences

Cognitive abilities seem to have a significant impact on adult learners and are divided into four categories:

1. Cognitive abilities

Two basic types of cognitive abilities are *fluid* intelligence, which is similar to traditional ideas of intelligence quotient (IQ) and refers to the ability to solve problems, and *crystallized* intelligence, which is a function of experience and education.

The implication of this research is that instructors must be alert to the possibility that adult learners, particularly older ones, may not respond as quickly to new material or situations and that adjustments must be made to allow additional time for learning. Conversely, when learning depends on prior experience and education, no adjustments should be needed because crystallized intelligence does not decrease until old age. However, fluid intelligence may. There are other multiple intelligences that have not yet been adequately measured.

2.   Cognitive controls

These patterns of thinking control ways individuals process and reason about information. They regulate perception and are direct descendants of cognitive abilities.

3.   Cognitive styles

Often, the terms *cognitive learning style* and *learning style* are erroneously used interchangeably. Cognitive styles are more stable traits and refer to the way a person gathers, organizes, and processes information.

Each individual brings various cognitive learning styles into the classroom. Students learn by one or a combination of methods:
- Visual learners learn by seeing or imaging.
- Auditory learners learn by listening and verbalizing.
- Tactile learners learn by touching and manipulating.

- Kinesthetic learners learn by doing and being involved.

The more senses an educator can appeal to, the more likely the information will be retained. An educator should try to appeal to as many of the senses as possible. If students hear it, see it, talk about it, and then do it, retention of the information is more effective.

For example, if an educator says to her class, "Take out the red book, and turn to chapter 24 and complete questions 1 through 4," and only provides verbal instructions, the visual learner will have difficulty understanding. If the educator writes the information on the board, saying nothing, the auditory learner will have difficulty processing the information. If the educator writes the information on the board, tells the class verbally, and then shows the students the red book, there will be a greater chance of students with various cognitive learning styles retaining the information.

4. Learning styles

Learning styles refer to the broadest range of how individuals learn. Kolb's model, the LSI learning inventory, suggests that individuals learn from feeling, observing, doing, and thinking, or a combination of methods. Other models used for measuring learning style dimensions are Gregorc, Canfield, Dunn & Dunn, Myers-Briggs, and Costa and McRae.

Personality

Personality includes attention and engagement styles, anxiety, and tolerance for unrealistic expectations, vagueness, and frustration. Personality also includes control, achievement, and risk-taking issues.

Prior Knowledge

Prior knowledge can be referred to as achievement or structural knowledge. It can be an asset or a liability. Changing a student's existing ideas is sometimes more difficult than teaching a student without prior knowledge. The instructor should start from the student's current level of knowledge. In each class, the instructor will encounter various levels of knowledge, and it helps to positively acknowledge the previous way of doing things.

Effective adult-learning professionals use their understanding of individual differences to tailor adult learning experiences in various ways. They apply core principles to fit the learners' cognitive abilities and learning style preferences. They use core principles to identify which of them are applicable to a specific group of learners. They use core principles to expand the goals of learning experiences.

2 The Adult Learning Process

What are the steps in the learning process?

The development, organization, and presentation of adult education programs require a continuous application of eight basic steps. These steps ensure that the framework, and several topics, such as formulating objectives, designing learning activities, and implementing and evaluating programs, are covered in depth in each section of the text applicable to them.

Learning can be stimulated or blocked by a variety of internal and external factors. The following eight steps may be viewed as a learning system model for addressing these factors and facilitating the learning process:

Step 1. Setting the climate for learning

Verbal and nonverbal messages

All types of messages are communicated to persons from the physical, human, and organizational environments in which they live or work. People become adept at picking up and decoding such messages, whether the signals are verbal or nonverbal. Unfortunately, those responsible for organizational structure, learning facilitation, and other components and activities of the workplace are not always aware of the meaning and power of such messages, especially the nonverbal type.

Organizational climates vary from warm and informal to dull and ego deflating.

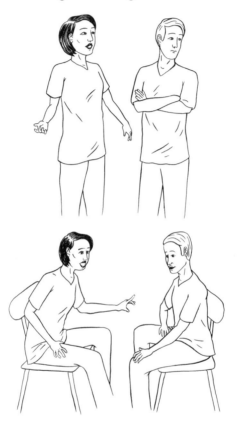

Physical surroundings

Physical surroundings are concerned with space, light, decor, temperature, comfort, seating arrangements, and refreshments. The nurse educator may have little control over the location and surroundings of where the class is conducted. Even so, the educator should attempt to make the classroom a place of learning and should initiate and improve on the items that one has control over. Make the room inviting by placing posters or pictures on the wall and adding flowers, a coffeepot, or a bowl of candy. Ensure that books and learning resources are available for reference and use.

Refreshments are preferred for in-service meetings, and nurse educators should budget for these items. Cookies and coffee are incentives for staff to attend, if only for the free food. Getting the staff there physically is half the battle. Most have heard the old saying, "You can lead a horse to water, but you can't make it drink." This may be true, but once it's there, you *can* make it thirsty.

Informal classroom seating arrangements work much better for adults than formal classroom seating. The typical, formal classroom seating with forward-facing seats tends to stifle communication and interaction among students. Students are unable to see the faces of anyone except the instructor. All they can see are the backs of the heads of the students in front of them. A U-shaped seating arrangement allows students to see the faces of all the other students, as well as the instructor. This arrangement promotes a greater exchange of information and ideas.

Interpersonal relationships

The nurse educator needs to create a climate of trust, respect, acceptance, openness, and a non-threatening attitude in the classroom. Many ways are open to the educator to interact with students for building a climate of trust and openness. The nurse educator's verbal and, especially, nonverbal communications set the tone of the classroom. The nurse educator should be tactful when correcting mistakes, taking care not to embarrass students. The educator's primary goal is to provide students with correct information and skills training. Mistakes are a normal part of learning. If students expect to be ridiculed or embarrassed, they will be reluctant to participate. A good educator creates conditions that guarantee frequent and early successes. Each success builds enthusiasm and leads to future successes.

The nurse educator should treat each student with respect. Be even-handed with praise, and give compliments for good answers or completed student projects.

The nurse educator needs to set clear goals. Let students know what is expected of them. The educator knows what will be taught; likewise, the students need to know what is going to be taught and what is expected of them. They should be clear on the educator's expectations by the end of the class, so they have an opportunity to know which elements and tasks to focus on. The educator should set behavioral objectives to the level of the class, and limit objectives to a reasonable amount, which can be accomplished in the allotted class time. Share the goals and objectives with the students, so everyone is working toward the same end.

Here are two examples that illustrate the nurse educator's approach to informing the class about goals and objectives:

"Today we will be covering chapter 25 in our textbook. We will be reviewing the material during the first part of class, and, during the second part of the class, you will be expected to complete a quiz on the material covered in chapter 25."

"At the end of this in-service, each of you will be expected to demonstrate the proper use of a fire extinguisher."

Step 2. Organization

Organizational preparation deals with policy, structure, theme, displays, budget, and frequency of activity. Be creative! Consider some of these ways to organize and announce training sessions:

- Post bright, funny, cartooned notices for in-service meetings.
- Advertise an afternoon in-service that includes popcorn and a movie.
- Select themes for meetings that coincides with a holiday or a national theme. If October is "National Fire Safety Month," what better time to present the annual fire safety in-service?

Schedule in-service programs at the same time and day each month, if possible and appropriate. In this manner, all staff members know, for example, that an in-service is conducted at 2:00 P.M on the second Monday of each month. This also allows supervisors to schedule staff for the meetings.

Develop a master education calendar. In scheduling the calendar, present required education material first; then, schedule the education for staff-development presentations. Divide staff-development in-services into two categories—skills development and human relation's development.

Remember that staff members require in-services on subjects other than skills alone. Subjects that will enrich the staff's personal development include such topics as communication, personal safety, team building, and problem solving. Remember to allow time for scheduling and developing needed in-services.

Step 3. Establishing a structure for mutual planning

Involving the learner is crucial to establishing a structure for mutual planning. Elicit the input of learner needs, interests, and values. Using information gathered in the needs assessment is helpful in this stage of planning. The educator can help establish a structure for mutual planning by actively involving the student in collaborative efforts and, also, by creating an environment of trust and nonthreatening openness and recognizing the student's right to make mistakes.

Step 4. Assessing needs, interests, and values

Prioritize and discuss the feasibility of needs, interests, and values of the staff. The educator's ideas concerning staff's needs and interests may be much different than the staff's perceived needs or the needs of administration.

Consider this example:

Administration and the staff developer have identified a problem in staff's understanding of an advance directive. The nurse educator makes a list of three to four topics for future in-services, one of which is "Understanding Advance Directives." The notice is given to all involved staff, and it asks them to choose the in-service topics they would like to have presented to them by checking the box next to the chosen topic and, also, ranking the topics in order of importance to them. When the completed notices are collected, the nurse educator presents the in-service on "Advance Directives." It is more acceptable to staff because, although they may not have ranked this topic as their first choice, they were given a choice. After presenting the "Advance Directive" in-service, the educator presents other suggested topics as time and schedule permit.

Step 5. Formulating objectives

Objectives must be realistic, attainable, and measurable. Behavioral objectives should answer four questions: Who? What behavior? Under what conditions? How well or to what degree of mastery is desired?

A well-constructed behavioral objective is measurable. The educator can then construct an evaluation tool of choice (test) using questions that meet the stated behavioral objectives.

Consider this example of a behavioral objective:

The student will be able to describe modifications needed for activities of daily living.

The test question related to this behavioral objective might be constructed as follows: "List three modifications needed for activities of daily living and describe the use of each."

Or, if the in-service topic is on body mechanics,

one of the behavioral objectives might be stated this way:

The student will be able to demonstrate two safe lifting techniques.

The verification that the stated behavioral objective was met may be in the form of a demonstration, or it may be answered by a test question—multiple choice or any other type of question, as long as it meets the stated behavioral objective of the information that was taught.

Step 6. Designing learning activities

Instead of using the content of someone else's program, the educator may wish to redesign or modify the program and use preferred training skills to assist others in achieving their own learning goals. Plan short learning steps. Do not pack too much information into a short period of time. More information is learned and retained if it is presented in small digestible portions.

The lesson plan is a designed learning activity. In other words, the lesson plan is an outline of what is to be presented. A lesson plan should contain the following seven elements:

- Topic
- Behavioral objectives
- Information to be presented
- Teaching methods to be employed
- Equipment needed (handouts, videos)
- Evaluation questions
- Required time frame

Describe three important facts about the interaction between dignity and caregiving

Estimated Time:
   10 minutes

Tools:
   Handout: Why is dignity so important?
   Transparency: Important ideas about dignity
   Video: Promoting Dignity–It's everyone's job!

Learning Activity: Discussion and Exercise

Make the following points:

All of us like to be treated with dignity. People in healthcare facilities do too.

Dignity and respect are something we should use in all our interactions with our residents and with whatever type of care we provide.

After distributing handout and displaying transparency ask the following question for discussion:

What parts of our residents' lives do we care for in this facility?

Make the following point:

Dignity touches all areas of care.

Step 7. Implementing learning activities

Promote active learning, not passive learning.
Passive learning is simply receiving information. It
includes listening or watching. Active learning is
participation by the student by actively doing
things such as working problems, trying new
skills, or hands-on activities.

Make learning fun! Use as many teaching methods
as possible. Use games, contests, and role-play for
learning experiences. A director of staff development shared her idea:

> She planned to burst into the classroom,
> dressed in bright red pajamas, carrying a fire
> bucket full of confetti for the usual, required
> ho-hum fire/safety in-service. Her idea was to
> get the students attention, and once she got
> their attention and created the interest, the next
> step would be to present the information.

Make the student want to be there. Be creative.
Give prizes for the most in-services attended.
Create the "Apple of the Month" award for a special
achievement. Start a contest to name the next
month's in-service, or develop a mascot for the
education department. Give out balloons, candy
bars, and other items for achievements. Everybody
likes a gift now and then, no matter how small.
These items make the learner remember what fun
they had.

Step 8. Evaluating learner activities

Evaluating the activity reveals to what degree the

student learned and how effective the educator has performed. Measurement of learning outcomes is documented by an evaluation mechanism designed to reflect the behavioral objectives as being met. An evaluation method can be documentation, observation, return demonstration, or written test. Evaluation of the program is the first step in the reassessment of the program.

Learning outcomes can be evaluated by many methods. Written tests are not always warranted. The type of learning outcome mechanism designed depends upon the level of the participants, course content, length of the program, and the preference of the educator.

Each program, in-service, learning experience, or nursing workshop should include behavioral objectives. They are usually presented as follows:

> By the end of this program the participant will be able to . . . (followed by a list of behavioral objectives).

Learning outcome measurements are created from the behavioral objectives. The presentation then meets the objectives set at the beginning of the program. To verify that learning occurred, the achievement of the stated objectives must be documented. For example, suppose the objective was stated in this way:

> The participant will be able to list two or three things learned today.

This is difficult to measure. If the behavioral objective was stated in this way:

> At the end of the presentation the participant will be able to correctly identify two of the major signs and symptoms of fluid overload.

The student's response to the question on the evaluation tool would meet the program behavioral objectives.

3 The Challenges of Staff Development

In any organization, there exists a hierarchy of purposes, philosophies, goals, and objectives. These purposes are incorporated into the job role of the nurse educator. Education in the acute hospital setting also includes educational requirements that must be met by the Joint Commission on Accreditation of Healthcare Organizations (JCAHO), OSHA, OBRA, and, in California, Title XXII guides the content of educational information required for long-term care facilities.

If nurse educators are to meet the major needs of hospital management, which includes being in compliance with federal and state regulations, minimizing employee turnover, and maximizing employee productivity, all levels of management must become involved.

This means that the staff development/education department cannot be expected to stand alone and that other levels of management should be involved in the education of the staff and work as a team in meeting the goals of the facility. Other challenges facing the nurse educator in an organized healthcare setting include the various levels and disciplines of employees requiring education, multiple areas of nursing specialties, and other multiple duties incorporated into the job description.

Essential Elements of Staff Development

The role of staff development contains two main elements—orientation and in-service/staff development programs.

Orientation programs are fairly standard in the content and topics presented, which include policies and procedures, philosophy of the organization, emergency, fire safety procedures, and an overall view of other departments and their functions.

Staff development includes required program topics plus various programs for maintaining staff competencies, morale, and problem resolution.

To create cost-effective, staff development/in-service programs for competencies or problem resolution, it is necessary to include these five critical elements:

1. Identifying the real problem

2. Designing an appropriate solution

3. Testing the solution

4. Revisiting that solution as necessary

5. Implementing and evaluating the results

All nurses in the organization should recognize that contributing to staff development and using systematic problem-solving processes is a natural part of their nursing practice. It is essential to ensure the competency of nursing practices and quality patient care. Analysis of the problem frequently reveals the need for a mixed approach to problem resolution, using both management as well as educational interventions.

Why are needs important in learning?

Every human being has needs. Maslow described in his hierarchy of needs the basic animal needs shared by everyone. Maslow theorized that as each need is met, a new set of needs emerge in order. After the basic physical needs, such as air, water, and necessities for life are satisfied, the next set of needs emerges: safety and security. Maslow also theorized that until these basic needs are met, the others are of no particular concern. Maslow's described set of needs continues with ego needs and, ultimately, reaches the self-actualization or fulfillment level.

Maslow's Hierarchy of Needs

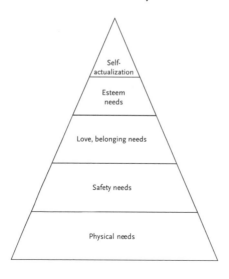

An unsatisfied need is a motivator. Physical needs, security needs, and the need to belong are fairly self-satisfied in today's society. Once an individual feels his self-esteem needs are essentially satisfied, the final set of needs emerge and are often referred to as fulfillment needs. Factors that motivate adults to learn can be life changes or the seeking of learning experiences in order to cope with specific life-changing events. Other factors may include increasing the learner's self-esteem or job enhancement. Adults need to be able to integrate new ideas into the ideas they already know, if they are going to keep and use the new information.

The astute educator can learn to recognize those needs and employ techniques that trigger motivation in the learner by planning programs around the needs and ranges of the learner. To accomplish this, an adequate needs assessment should be performed.

"Investigate before you educate" is old and practical guidance. A needs approach is the first step in planning learning experiences. The perceived needs of management may not be the perceived needs of the staff. This approach is significantly different from simply prescribing a program and providing new information to adults without attempting to identify and meet learners' true needs.

What is a need?

A need is a gap or discrepancy between current outcomes and required, desired, or specified outcomes.

What is a needs assessment?

A needs assessment defines the desired outcome, determines the validity of educational program objectives, and bridges the gap between current outcomes and desired results. It helps focus on the end instead of the means.

A needs assessment ordinarily consists of three fundamental elements:

1. Identifying that there is a "gap" to be closed

2. Considering alternate ways and means to close the gap

3. Avoiding selecting the solution before the problems are really known, implement acceptable solutions

Planning a Needs Assessment

In conducting a needs assessment, the educator should first consider the student's physiological and psychological requirements, as well as process requirements and task requirements that the student is able to perform. The expressed needs of the student should also be considered. The educator can ascertain what information, understanding, feelings, attitudes, and skills would be adequate for developing designated behavioral objectives in program development or in problem resolution. There is also value to a needs assessment approach in problem solving. Some problems may warrant simultaneous interventions among multiple departments and services.

Needs-assessment information on task and process requirements may be gathered from several data sources:

- Policy noncompliance
- Standardized test scores
- Direct personal observation
- Survey results
- Analysis statistics
- Personal interviews
- Staff input
- Critical incidents
- Quality assurance (QA) reports
- Risk management assessments

Assessment material from employees regarding their perceived educational needs may be in the form of a questionnaire. The questionnaire should list no more than three selected choices, and the employees should rank them in order of importance. The employee may be asked to write in a suggested topic. The information gathered will give the educator a sense of what the employees view as important. Allowing employees to suggest topics that are of value to them gives them a feeling of inclusiveness and a sense of commitment.

An effective needs assessment is useful in developing objectives toward educational outcomes. The total program can then be properly directed and can assist all educational partners to focus on the ends rather than the means. Generally, adults participate voluntarily in educational programs, thus making it extremely important that participants see the program as directly related to their needs. If the program is viewed by the participants as not being helpful to them, there will be little interest or participation. To maintain program relevance to the participant, the nurse educator should avoid hasty conclusions, actions, or activities that will expend resources needlessly and not result in effective problem resolution.

Is the problem one that staff development can resolve?

Historically, hospital administration has operated under the impression that if a problem arises anywhere within the facility, presenting an in-service program will immediately correct the problem.

If a problem is identified, the educator should ask these four basic questions before spending time and effort on an in-service about problem solving:

1. Is there evidence of staff member's lack of skill or knowledge?

2. Is it clear that other departments or services are meeting their obligations and performing their prescribed functions?

3. Are policies and procedures adequate for the situation?

4. Does the problem disappear when a skilled staff member performs the task or function?

These questions elicit responses that will lead to a shared implementation of a needs approach. Remember: needs are not fixed; they are constantly changing.

46

4 Role of the Educator

In addition to applying the eight steps of the learning process presented in chapter 3, the role of the educator encompasses such responsibilities as being a change agent and facilitating communication in the learning process. Clarity was also mentioned as one of the primary characteristics and skills needed by educators for motivating learners. The educator is a facilitator and does not necessarily need to be an expert in all content knowledge to guide the process effectively, but the educator must possess good communication skills.

The Educator as Communicator

Communication is the exchange of thoughts, ideas, information, and attitudes by verbal and nonverbal means. Communication is a *two-way* process that involves the sending and receiving of information.

Nursing professionals often get stuck in *one-way* communication. One-way communication eliminates the feedback created when the receiver of the message responds. One-way communication is quicker, faster, and saves an enormous amount of time. It can be easily identified in such phrases as, "Sit up," "Roll over," or, "Take this pill." One-way communication sounds more like a command and leaves little chance for feedback or response of the receiver. This type of communication is necessary in certain emergency situations. One certainly

48

wouldn't ask someone's opinion about giving epi-
nephrine in a code situation or schedule a confer-
ence about a fire in the cafeteria.

Two-way communication gives the receiver an
opportunity to respond and verify the message and
send a response to the sender. Here are two examples:

> Sender: "Mrs. Porter, are you able to sit up to
> take your medication?"
>
> Receiver: "Yes."
>
> Sender: "Do you see a problem in having your
> term paper completed by Friday?"
>
> Receiver: "No."

Communication is intended to involve the receiver,
who then sends a communication back to the
sender.

Verbal communication is any sound, including a
word, cry, groan, or a scream. It uses only one of
our senses, hearing. Nonverbal communication
uses other senses: sight, smell, and touch. Touch is
a strong nonverbal communicator; a touch can
communicate much more than words. Silence is
another commanding nonverbal communication,
one often forgotten. Long silences at appropriate
times can be a very effective method of communication. Seventy percent of human communication
is communicated by nonverbal means. Humans
are quick at reaching conclusions based upon
another's actions. Attitudes, values, and emotions

are communicated more clearly by one's gestures, walk, dress, expressions, and behavior than through the spoken word.

Nurses are normally adept at using their powers of observation because they routinely observe and assess the total patient/client. For example, if a nurse asks a patient whether she is in pain, and the patient replies, "No," while grimacing and holding her side, the nurse instinctively uses her observation abilities to reach a conclusion. In a classroom situation, the instructor's nonverbal communication "speaks louder" than verbal communication.

General Barriers to Communication

Communication is an important part of teaching. Recognizing existing, basic human barriers in the communication process will better assist the educator in providing clarity and understanding for students. There are many barriers to communication, four of which are briefly described here:

Failure to listen

Failure to listen can be caused by both internal and external factors.

Internal

It is difficult to listen when one is experiencing internal factors such as fear, anger, worry, fatigue, family problems, financial problems, or a number of other stress factors. Physical impairment, pain, or hearing problems also affect listening.

External

External conditions involve such elements as noise, temperature, time, location, comfort, and surroundings. As examples, students do not listen well if it is past lunch time or end of class time, when the classroom temperature is either too cold or to warm, or when they are in some way uncomfortable. The instructor has some control over external conditions. For good listening conditions, one may reduce outside noise, select the proper temperature of the classroom, provide breaks at frequent intervals, and maintain class schedules.

Language

This barrier to communication may be caused by differences of vocabulary, language, or dialect. Medical terms, many of which are in Latin, can be intimidating and create a barrier. Medical terms are difficult to understand; medical jargon is a language all its own. Instead of asking a patient/client if she has been NPO, it would be more appropriate to ask, "What did you eat or drink since midnight?"

Selective hearing

People hear what they wish to hear. In other words, they shut out what is unpleasant, choosing to ignore what is being said. A patient/client who is told by his physician to give up cigarettes and start to exercise at least two times a week selectively chooses to hear only the part about the exercise.

The educator needs to give clear instructions when giving assignments, as in this example:

Vocabulary words are due on Monday. Does anyone foresee a problem with having them in by Monday?

Failure to check assumptions

Failure to check assumptions is ingrained in nurses in nursing school, but failure to check assumptions also applies to the communication process. Never assume the other party understands what has been said.

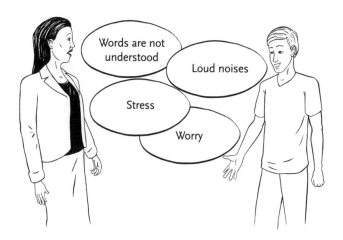

Why is communication in a health facility challenging?

Even under ideal conditions, communication can be difficult. In social situations, if one wants to communicate effectively, the best possible surroundings are selected, preferably in a comfortable, relaxed, quiet atmosphere. A time is chosen that is convenient to the listener, and then communication proceeds.

Barriers to communication (described previously) exist in healthcare settings. Classrooms may be far from ideal in comfort, temperature, or noise level. The time for class presentations may not be conducive for communication. The nurse educator who attempts to teach students who are hungry, fatigued, or under stress; who may have difficulty understanding the language or medical terms; or who are in an uncomfortable environment can conclude the learning process may be affected.

Listening

Listening can be dynamic, like listening to a concert. Listening is sometimes the better part of communication, if done purposefully and intelligently. Listening may be considered the highest form of communicating. Public and private learning institutions present courses on the subjects of writing, reading, and speaking, but few on listening. Good listening habits are taught, not caught.

Good listening involves judging the *content* of the message not only its *delivery*. Whether a sentence is spoken in halting broken phrases or delivered in a perfect Oxford accent does not guarantee that the content is true. When taking a medical history, one listens "between the lines" for what the patient/client is not saying.

In general, adults can speak 125 words per minute but understand 450 words per minute; therefore, a "thought-lag" exists, where the listener's thoughts naturally go wandering off. *This is the major reason why teaching by lecture alone is one of the most ineffective methods of teaching.*

Suggestions for Good Listening

- Stop talking: listening starts when you stop talking.
- Put the speaker at ease by using open body language.
- Show you are listening by looking at the speaker.
- Try to hear what is being said, rather than how it is being said.
- Empathize with the speaker.
- Be patient; allow ample time for listening.
- Keep an open mind.
- Try to see things from the speakers point of view.
- Ask questions; paraphrase the speaker.

A popular saying is, "Nature gave man two ears but only one tongue," a gentle reminder that we should listen more than we talk.

The Educator as an Agent of Change

The role of the staff educator involves many changes. In actuality, training is all about change. The introduction of new knowledge changes in procedures, policy, regulations, or all of them inclusively. Change is always occurring.

When is change acceptable? Planning is filled with observations concluding that human nature resists change. Like most generalities, this is only partially true. People welcome some changes.

The educator's objective is to make small changes that seem desirable to most everyone involved. Below are guidelines to assist the educator when

initiating change—any change—to benefit employees and students:

- Change presents a fear of the unknown.
- Change is more acceptable when the reason for
  the change is explained thoroughly and is understood.
- Change is more acceptable when it does not
  threaten security.
- Change is more acceptable when those affected
  by it have helped to create it.
- Change is more acceptable when based on previous knowledge and experience.
- Change is more acceptable when it follows a
  series of successful changes.
- Change is more acceptable when not instituted
  during other major changes.
- Change is more acceptable if it has been planned
  and not unexpected.
- Change is more acceptable to new employees
  than those who have been on the job a long period of time.
- Change is more acceptable to people who will
  share in the benefits.
- Change is more acceptable to people who have
  been trained to plan for change.

It is critical that, for any change, the reasons for
implementing the change be communicated clearly
to those who will be affected, whether positively or
negatively.

The Educator as a Conflict Manager

The educator assumes many roles and, much like any other managerial position, will encounter conflict. Common sources of conflict include differences stemming from incompatible perceptions of information, overly functional responsibility, and authority. In other words, conflict occurs when the involved parties believe that what each wants is incompatible with what others want. Conflicts often arise over these areas:

- Facts
- Goals
- Roles
- Methods
- Values
- Needs

Conflict can be easily analyzed by asking two key questions:

What is the nature of our differences?

What may be the reasons for our differences?

Guidelines in Diagnosing Conflict

Conflict is an inevitable and important process. Conflicts are likely to increase in a time of change. Conflict, like any other human process, can produce both positive and negative results.

Negative aspects of conflict
- People feel defeated.
- Climate of distrust and suspicion may develop.

- Emotional distance may increase between those involved.

Positive aspects of conflict

- New ideas are generated.
- Problems emerge and are resolved.
- Tension of conflict stimulates interest.

Identifying Conflict Styles

The nurse educator will probably encounter conflicts with students, managers, administration, and other staff members. Identifying the administrative conflict style and identifying when the appropriate use of a particular style is needed may assist the nurse educator toward productive, individual and system-type conflict resolution.

Individuals develop characteristic styles they use in conflict situations. Often, individuals develop two or three typical responses to a situation, depending on the degree of conflict. Each type of conflict style is appropriate in a given situation. Many conflict styles develop from family, social, or life experiences of the individual.

Organizations or systems often develop a typical conflict style in management. Sometimes organizations can become frozen in a particular conflict style.

The model identifying five conflict styles, as described by Kilman and Thomas (1975), are still cited and of great value:

1. Competitive (assertive and uncooperative)

This style is appropriate when a quick, conclusive decision is needed, as in emergencies, on issues where one is certain of a particular position, or issues in which an unpopular course of action must be implemented. This style is power oriented and usually refers to pursuing one's own concerns at the expense of others.

2. Collaboration (assertive and cooperative)

This style is more effective in finding an integrative solution when both sets of concerns are too important to be compromised, and to merge insights from people with different perspectives.

3. Compromising (intermediate assertive and cooperative)

This conflict style is used when goals are moderately important but not worth the effort or potential disruption of more assertive roles. It may be used effectively when two opponents with equal power are strongly committed to mutually exclusive goals, as in labor-management bargaining.

4. Avoiding (unassertive and uncooperative)

This style should be used only when an issue is trivial or when the potential damage of confronting a conflict outweighs the benefits of its resolution. It also may be used when the nurse educator has no power or chance of satisfying concerns and may be viewed as a form of diplomacy.

5.   Accommodating (unassertive and cooperative)

This style is used when one realizes one is wrong, to demonstrate that one is reasonable, or when an issue is much more important to another. This style may also be used to build up social credits for later issues of more importance or when perceived harmony and avoiding disruption is especially important.

5 Constructing Objectives

An objective is a measurable step toward an identified goal and identifies who will accomplish a specific task, as well as the means for accomplishing
the task. Specific or behavioral objectives will identify to what degree and under what conditions it
will be met.

Teaching presentations contain both content and
process objectives. The content objectives or
instructional objectives include both the information, concepts, theories, ways of thinking, values,
and other substances that one can be expected to
learn which may also be termed as teaching outcomes. The general content is what is to be presented or to be learned by the student. Objectives
for learning should be designed to address three
major domains of learning objectives listed below.

Healthcare employees need knowledge skills, affective skills, and psychomotor skills to perform their
job roles adequately. Objectives for learning should
be designed to address the major domains in
which individuals learn. The field of nursing
encompasses three major domains of learning
objectives:

1. Cognitive domain (thinking)

This domain refers to designing objectives that are
concerned with how basic knowledge or information is learned and stored. Examples of objective

words in this domain: identify, choose, describe, select, classify, list, answer, and write.

2. Affective domain (feeling)

This domain considers behaviors relating to feelings, emotions, values, and needs. It is the most intangible portion of the learning process because individuals view events from different perspectives. Examples of affective terms: characterize, compare, contrast, differentiate, evaluate, analyze, conclude, assess, and interpret.

3. Psychomotor domain (doing)

This domain refers to designing objectives to facilitate the learning of a new procedure or skill and deals with the skills requiring the use and coordination of skeletal muscles. Examples of psychomotor terms: demonstrate, perform, give, place, use, show, present, draw, and make.

Teaching presentations include two kinds of objectives—content (instructional) objectives and process (specific, behavioral) objectives (or learning outcomes).

Content objectives, or general instructional objectives, are commonly associated with the term *goal* and can serve the important functions of establishing the broad framework for curriculum content planning and may be open to many interpretations. A content objective is a broad statement that reflects the desired outcome and does not contain reference-specific means. A content objective/goal describes an intended learning outcome for each subject taught. Each educator must define his or her own instructional objectives in terms of specific learning outcomes targeted for the learning level of each discipline. Content objectives includes these components:

- Information
- Concepts
- Theories
- Ways of thinking
- Values
- Other substance that one can be expected to learn, also called teaching outcomes

Here is an example of a content objective:

> At the end of this session, the student will be able to describe diagnostic tests for respiratory disorders.

After the educator selects a content objective for the planned lesson, specific or behavioral objectives are developed. Within the general content objective or learning outcome should be the specific behavioral objectives the student is expected to learn. The number of specific objectives/process objectives may vary according to the length of the planned lesson in order to adequately evaluate learning outcome.

Process objectives measure the student's learning. These objectives need to be written in sequential order to lead to a logical learning experience. The procedure for defining instructional objectives in behavioral terms should include these four basic components: who, what, how well, and to what degree.

The nurse educator should ask the following questions when writing behavioral objectives. (As a learning aid, remember these components in their alphabetical order):

Audience

Who is the audience? Always the student.

Behavior

What will the student learn? This question identifies what observable or measurable behavior the student is expected to demonstrate. Each specific objective starts with a verb that indicates observable or measurable behavior.

Identify the action verb. Follow the action verb with a content reference that describes the subject, such as name, discuss, make, perform, and list.

For example:

> *Name* is the action verb; *body systems* is a content reference.

Here are a few more examples:

> Demonstrate: hand washing

> Make: an occupied bed

> Identify: basic rules of safety

> Assemble: the items necessary for

Conditions

Under what conditions (restrictions or parameters) will learning be identified?

Look at these examples:

Without the aid of the textbook

Using a specific diagram

Degree

How well will the student demonstrate the degree of mastery? Identify acceptable competency or performance. Include a performance standard that indicates to what degree of outcome is acceptable:

80% out of 100%

3 out of 4

Wrinkle free

Within the allotted time frame

Other, as appropriate

Here are two examples, as described to the student before the student begins the lesson:

At the end of this session, the student will be able to calculate I.V. drip rates. (This defines only who and what, and is open to interpretation.)

Given two examples, the student will correctly calculate from memory the I.V. drip rates. (This defines who, what, how, and to what degree of mastery.)

The number of behavioral objectives is determined by the content to be covered, the time frame of the presentation, the learning styles of the students, and the complexity of the materials. There should be a clear link between the level of objective and the level of learning of the student. The educator cannot expect the nursing assistant to meet behavioral objectives that use terms and activities that are likely beyond their educational and experiential level, such as these:

- Compare and contrast
- Distinguish between
- Hypothesize
- Interpret

When training nursing assistants, these cognitive and psychomotor descriptive terms may be more appropriate to use:

- Assemble
- Choose
- Demonstrate
- Find List
- List
- Name
- Perform
- Pick
- Place
- Select
- Show
- State

Test questions should be constructed from the behavioral objectives. The test (evaluation tool) documents that the behavioral objectives for the presentation were met. *Note that evaluation tools are not always in written form.*

Carefully constructed behavioral objectives will be

the educator's simple guide to constructing effective evaluation tools that adequately measure learning outcomes. Keep in mind that the more objectives constructed, the more test questions must be constructed and included.

The following list will assist the educator in selecting the appropriate descriptive words for behavioral objectives. Behavioral objectives usually use action verbs. The educator should *avoid* the use of behavioral objective terms that are difficult to measure or evaluate, such as these examples:

- The learner will *appreciate* the value of...
- ...understand
- ...realize
- ...know
- ...become familiar with
- ...comprehend
- ...become aware of
- ...realize
- ...develop an understanding of

In contrast, these examples of cognitive or psychomotor descriptive terms may be more appropriate.

The learner will be able to *name* two or more characteristics of dehydration.

Given a list of symptoms, the student will *identify* those directly related to Paget's disease by circling the symptom.

List three of the most common sites in which cancer occurs in women.

6 Creating An Effective Lesson Plan

Lesson plans are, essentially, maps or outlines intended to assist the educator with important components of the presentation. These include the sequence of events to be presented, the time allotted for each topic, content information, materials, and evaluation methods.

The following list is a useful guideline for preparing lesson plans:

1. Select a specific topic to be taught in one session.

2. Determine the objectives, and state them in measurable behavioral terms.

3. List specific subtopics.

4. Maintain continuity in the sequence of events by listing topics in order and presenting information in a logical, sequential order.

5. State methods of instruction to be used.

6. Describe instructional activities in sufficient detail, to be able to teach from the lesson plan.

7. List all necessary materials and teaching aids.

8. Develop the evaluation tool/testing mechanism.

9. Reevaluate the time frame for the lesson.

Lesson Plan Format

A properly prepared lesson plan should be sufficiently descriptive, in outline form, to allow anyone to teach from it. It will save the educator valuable time because, once a lesson plan has been developed, it can be filed away for repeated use, until the material needs requires updating or renewal. Although the basic plan is in place, the educator may wish to make slight modifications, depending on the group, student needs, or change in procedure.

The following sections are presented as a standard format for preparing lesson plans:

- Behavioral objectives (realistic measurable, attainable)
- Materials needed (physical materials and resources, e.g., videos and overheads)
- Presentation material (specific information to be taught and time frame, in sequential order)
- Instructional methods (lecture, overhead, handouts, demonstration, role-play, group learning, or other method to be employed)
- Evaluation/test (questions are constructed from the behavioral objectives, which can be measured with written test questions, skills checklist, or direct observation, as decided by the educator)

Consider these examples:

Behavioral objective

The student will be able to list three common therapeutic measures used for the incontinent patient/client.

Evaluation question options

List three common therapeutic measures used for the incontinent patient/client.

Given a list of therapeutic measures used for the incontinent patient/client, circle three of the most common methods used. (Note: The evaluation question may be constructed in a form that is more easily completed by the student and easier to correct by the educator.)

A copy of the completed lesson plan, evaluation tool, and sign-in sheet must be retained in the educator's files. If a guest speaker is presenting, the speaker's résumé or list of qualifications must be included, as well as the speaker's lesson plan with objectives.

Note: More extensive material on test construction is discussed in chapters 9 and 10.

70

7 Steps in the Teaching Process

Five-Step Teaching Process

The five-step teaching process is simple, direct, and provides an analytical method of organizing of the art of teaching. This process is of the utmost importance in a nursing school setting.

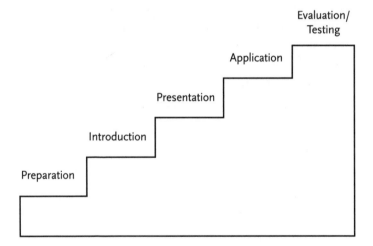

Step 1. Preparation

Preparation is the first and most important step of teaching. This is where the educator uses the lesson plan. Simply stated, set clear goals, have materials on hand, plan short steps of learning, and schedule sufficient time.

In preparing the lesson, the educator must not forget to prepare the learner. Motivation is probably the most important condition for learning. If the student is not ready to learn, the educator cannot force the student to learn.

In job-related classes, most students recognize the connection between what they learn and what they earn. The educator should make every effort to create an atmosphere that motivates the learner.

Step 2. Introduction

The educator needs to create an interest and a need for learning. A good introduction is the most important part of any presentation. Within the introduction, the educator can use great amounts of creative imagination to get the students' attention and interest and create an incentive for them to listen. The introduction must appeal to the individual students' learning styles (refer to chapter 1).

A good introduction should create interest and motivation by

- demonstrating interesting and useful applications of the new knowledge (e.g., save time, reduce work load, improve skills, etc.)
- relating stories about the topic
- showing how the material presented will enhance the employee's job

Remember to share your enthusiasm. Ask questions designed to show that this information and/or skill is really needed.

Step 3. Presentation

Learning is an active process. Teaching is not merely telling.

- Incorporate audiovisual materials into the presentation.
- Vary teaching methods.
- If lecturing, vary the tempo, and ask questions of the students.
- Problem solve with the students: question, and answer questions.

Remember that students must participate in the learning process for learning to take place.

Step 4. Application

Practice is one of the most effective means of learning. Have students practice using the new material. Practice can be accomplished in many ways:
- discussing
- doing
- group activities
- return demonstration
- role-playing

Remember to give students opportunities to practice and correct mistakes before testing.

Step 5. Evaluation/Testing

Evaluations and tests are methods of measurement to verify what has been learned. They may be accomplished through a variety of mechanisms or activities:
- written
- oral
- problem solving
- return demonstration

In any organized educational experience there must be some type of verification or documentation that actual learning took place; this is what real education is all about. This is the critical factor that separates education and learning experiences from information just being presented. An evaluation tool documents that students have received and understood the information. The evaluation tool also tells the educator how well the lesson was taught.

The evaluation verifies that the learner heard, participated, and learned. Learning is similar to the communication process, in which sending, receiving, decoding, and resending are necessary to complete the communication cycle. Evaluation of what has been presented must be documented in some way.

Teaching without an evaluation tool is like shaking the feathers out of a feather pillow in a high wind: the educator has no quantifiable way of knowing how far the feathers went, who picked up the feathers, or if any were picked up at all.

The Learning Manager

Nurse educators need to be learning managers. Teachers are trained to be learning managers; they have been taught how to create effective learning conditions, both physical and psychological. Students are similar to computers: the instructor is responsible for entering the data into the "computer" and knowing the proper buttons to push to start the student problem-solving process.

The educator is a learning manager. A learning manager is similar to being a manager of a department in that the employees, like students, bring varying degrees of motivation, ability, attitude, and prior learning experiences with them. A learning manager also acts as a catalyst, managing conditions for learning:

Guide; don't push.

Each student is an individual who learns through various methods at an individualized pace. Set teaching goals that each student can attain.

Set rules.

Good rules are based on common sense and are time savers for the educator. To manage the classroom, the educator needs to set and discuss clear, sensible classroom rules about critical learning factors:

- punctuality
- absences
- break times
- testing procedures
- cell phone use
- recorders
- clean-up procedures

The educator should consider the consequences of each rule prior to the class.

The educator should refrain from making too many rules because every rule that is broken creates an enforcement problem; if the educator cannot enforce some of the rules, the educator sends the message that none of the rules need be taken seriously.

A basic rule about rules is that people will find a way to break rules they do not like. Each new rule will create a new behavior in the classroom. For example, if the educator tells the class that there will be no breaks, they may bring food and drink into the classroom, thus creating yet another problem.

Here is a list of basic rules that can help the educator stay focused and effective:

Arrive on time and start on time.

This rule sends the message to the students that the educator values the importance of the class.

Keep class discussions on track.

Facilitating is an important role in teaching. Avoid letting the more vocal students control the discussion.

Avoid public confrontations.

A public confrontation in the classroom usually results in a lose-lose situation for both educator and student. To turn it into a win-win situation, the educator should ask the student to step outside to discuss the differences and ask the student why he or she feels this way. Listen to the student, and try to arrive at a mutual agreement. If the situation cannot be quickly resolved, schedule an appointment after class to discuss the issue in more detail.

Facility managers usually have guidelines for dealing with conflict; it is wise to follow these guidelines.

8 Basic Instruction Methods

Most educators use a wide variety of instructional methods, according to the size and type of class, their subject, and the degree of teaching ability. A frequent change of pace will keep the class alert and active. The more senses appealed to while teaching, the better will adults learn. If learners see it, hear it, write it, and practice it, the material presented will be retained to a greater degree.

Lectures

Advantage: provides knowledge beyond textbook.

Disadvantage: provides passive learning.

Lectures should not continue beyond 15 minutes until the pace is changed. The educator may show overheads, stop to ask questions, explain how certain ideas and laws were discovered, and explain a related subject that is not in the textbook. The educator should not read from the text; students can do that themselves.

Florence Nightingale warns:

> You are not teaching skills or knowledge. You are teaching people. You must speak their language.

To improve the lecture, the educator should explain points not adequately covered in the text. In addition, the educator may relate personal nursing experiences that illustrate key points, use real-life examples to show how textbook information is actually applied, and explain how certain ideas were discovered.

During the lecture, the educator should look for confused looks among the students or stop and ask questions of the students. Think of a lecture as a conversation with a purpose. Interact with the students by asking questions that evoke responses of opinions, new ideas, values, and problem solving; this fosters critical thinking.

The educator may give the students clues during the lecture, such as these comments:

This is a test question.

You must know this equation from memory.

Finally, an educator should try not to lecture past the ending time of class. Listening usually ceases at that time.

Guest Speakers

Advantage: provides specialized knowledge.

Disadvantage: provides passive learning.

The educator should always review the subject with the guest speaker before the presentation. Prior to the guest speaker's presentation, the educator should give the speaker a specific time frame in which to present the subject, class level of understanding, and goals and objectives to be covered.

Student Presentation

Advantage: can increase student learning and participation.

Disadvantage: can be time consuming.

The educator should set a reasonable time limit for each presentation. The most positive aspect of this type of presentation is that students tend to learn from peers, and it keeps the class attention level high. This is also an excellent way for students to learn how to present information to others.

Discussion

Advantages: all students are involved, and it sparks new ideas.

Disadvantage: may be dominated by a few.

Discussion takes careful preparation. The educator should decide on a subject, with input from students. The educator should make a checklist of topics to be covered. The educator, who is the facilitator, should avoid giving an opinion but keep the group directed and focused.

In a classroom discussion, the educator is the monitor. If the class is large, the educator can divide the class into groups for discussion and guard against letting a few students dominate the discussion. To accomplish this, the educator should employ ways to involve those who have not participated. For example:

> Ask questions of students who are not actively participating, and involve them in the discussion.

Acknowledge the more vocal leaders of the discussion for their opinions, and then say, "Lets hear some opinions from some of the other students." After a brief pause, and if no one volunteers, the educator should then call on several students by name for their comments.

Make a summary on the blackboard of what the group agrees upon.

Questioning

Advantage: encourages participation.

Disadvantage: using closed questions (for yes or no responses) can limit higher order of thinking.

The educator should avoid using only closed questions because they limit higher orders of thinking. For example, instead of asking, "Is this drawing right?", the educator could ask, "What would you add to this drawing?"

Here are some examples of questions the educator might ask:

What would you do differently the next time?

How would you rate the quality of your work on this project?

Where do you think this needs improvement?

Why does this method work?

What is a better way to do it?

What did you do, and why?

What would happen if this step were left out?

The skilled educator does not ask, "Are there any questions?" Students will rarely respond; it is a yes or no question. If a student had a question or a point to be clarified, he or she might be hesitant to ask, not wanting to appear to be the only one in the class who did not understand. Worse still is asking that same question at the end of class time or past the end of class time; this discourages questions from the class because the students want to get out of class on time.

To be clear, the educator can ask open and closed types of questions. Some questions require only one correct answer, such as, "Can anyone tell me how many bones are in the hand?" Now, consider this question that the instructor is asking the class: "Why do you think this method works?"; this is an appropriate open-ended question.

Plan questions carefully. The best method for questioning a class is to ask the question of the entire class, pause, and then direct the question to one student by name. This method causes the entire class to consider the answer because they may be called upon for the answer. The educator should use questions to encourage shy students. If a student doesn't seem to know the answer, the educator should answer for the student, so the student is allowed to ease out of the uncomfortable situation while preserving his or her dignity. The educator may also provide clues to the student being questioned.

Simulation

Advantage: provides active learning.

Disadvantage: practice on models is less challenging than on real patients/clients.

Students pretend or imitate procedures performed on teaching models or other students. Simulation works well with students who are learning a skill. Learning takes place by doing as well as by observation.

Role-play

Advantages: increases problem-solving ability, and learning comes from peers.

Disadvantage: few students participate.

Role-play situations should be carefully planned. The educator should select the students carefully, choosing not only students who are outgoing, but those who do not readily participate.

It is beneficial in teaching interaction situations between patient/client and nursing personnel. Learning comes from several sources: students who role-play get the experience of dealing with others to problem solve while the rest of the class learns from observation. The greatest benefit comes from the discussion that follows.

Individualized Instruction

Advantage: students learn at their own pace.

Disadvantage: can be time consuming, working with students on a one-to-one basis with no interaction with other students.

This type of instruction is better accomplished in

an academic setting that has resources to tutor students.

Learning Packets/Self-Directed Instruction

Advantage: reduces classroom teaching time.

Disadvantage: provides passive learning.

Learning packets work well when a skill is being taught. They are used increasingly in hospital education orientation.

They are often developed to address only one level of learning, which makes the understanding of the information difficult for some students and unchallenging for others. Some students learn better through learning modalities other than reading. Learning packets do not allow for questions or interactions with the educator. Further, the instructor cannot easily verify whether students complete the work themselves, and some students may lack the motivation to work independently.

If learning packets are used, the educator should carefully prepare them with the same design concepts as classroom learning.

Demonstration

Advantage: provides active and passive learning.

Disadvantage: generally, none.

If the demonstration is performed correctly, it can be very effective in showing what happens; or, the educator may have students demonstrate the correct procedure to the class. Students tend to pay closer attention to classmates, and performing the demonstration gives students hands-on experience to reinforce concepts. It is very effective for skills learning.

Visual Media

Advantages: clarifies the subject and appeals to the visual learner.

Disadvantages: provides passive learning, and all media are not of equal standard or value.

Overhead transparencies can be used for choosing and controlling information to be shown to the class. The educator should arrange the room to be able to face the class while showing transparencies. The projector should be switched off until the transparency is ready to view and turned off when finished, to shift students' attention back to the instructor.

Use the "striptease" method for showing transparencies with more than one item on them, such as transparencies displaying lists. The striptease method of showing a transparency is simple: a plain piece of paper covers all of the transparency except the first item the educator wishes the student to view and focus on. As the discussion progresses and various points are covered, the educator moves the paper, exposing the next item to be discussed. Displaying the entire overhead containing points of interest arranged in list form tends to scatter the students' thought, and, while lecturing on the first item, the student may be reading and thinking about other items on the list.

Slides

Slides are effective for showing important points of a lecture, if they are done carefully and in sequence.

Videos

The educator should view the video before showing it to the students, if it is going to be used as a teaching tool. The educator should inform the students of the length of the video. Because videos provide passive learning experiences, the educator should make the class aware what is expected of them after viewing the video. Here are some suggestions:

"Look for three key points in this video that best describe..."

"Watch for the differences in how they manage..."

"Be ready to give a summary of..."

A discussion period should always follow a video presentation. It is best not to leave the room during the video presentation; this is not an excuse for a break or to use the video as a "baby-sitter" while completing other duties outside the classroom.

A lengthy video presentation should not be presented after an hour-long lecture; students attention span may be diminished. Showing a video presentation soon after lunch is also a poor choice of timing. Present the video after a short break, so students are refreshed and ready to focus.

Charts and Models

Charts, models, and other visuals can be effective teaching aids.

Computer-Assisted Instruction

Advantage: provides both passive and active learning.

Disadvantage: Little interaction with instructor.

This is an excellent source of learning. Facilities with large budgets are producing their own interactive programs for employees. *PowerPoint®* presentations for classes are the optimum of visual and didactic learning presentations.

All facilities may not have the capability of producing their own media, and it may be difficult to find packaged programs that apply to specific patient populations or that are congruent with standards and policies of individual facilities.

Gaming

Advantages: provides passive and active learning and creates competition, which stimulates motivation.

Disadvantage: generally, none.

Gaming is an effective method of instruction for individual and group problem-solving situations. Creative educators have latitude to develop many effective methods to stimulate student learning. Developing a crossword skill game on the blackboard, a *Jeopardy®*-type game, or even a million-

aire game sparks interest. Winning can be
achieved by accumulating points, and a small prize
can be awarded to winners. The educator is limited
only by his or her imagination.

9 Rationale for Testing

Tests should be used as teaching tools, not "road blocks" to learning. Tests should reinforce important points and concepts in the learning process, and should be designed to reflect the degree to which the objective is met.

Testing should be performed for these reasons:

Check student learning

Testing shows how far the class and the individual student is progressing in relation to stated objectives and provides feedback to the student about his or her progress.

Check for effective teaching

"If the student hasn't learned, then the teacher hasn't taught" is an old but true saying. The goal of the educator is to teach to pass, not to fail. If the majority of the group does poorly on a test, the educator should revise the test material or reevaluate the teaching methods.

Motivate students

Testing at regular intervals increases the student's motivation to study.

Grading purposes

Testing is an aid in assigning grades to students for their progress.

Types of Test Questions

The educator decides which type of information to obtain from the students by the type of test questions developed. If the information is vital and must be memorized, then recall questions should be employed.

- Recall – involves memorizing information.
- Recognition – requires the student to know something when viewed.
- Problem solving – requires the student to use both recall and recognition.
- Performance – requires the student to demonstrate learned skills.

Keeping Tests Fair and Objective

Objective test: answers are either right or wrong, making it difficult for the educator to be unfair or biased.

Subjective test: requires the educator to make judgments, and grading may be influenced by personal biases.

Types of Tests

Oral

An oral test is useful for students who have difficulty in reading comprehension. When asking questions in class, the educator is performing informal oral testing. Oral tests are not as objective as written tests. They must follow these guidelines:

- The educator should have the questions written down, so the same question is asked to all students the same way.
- Record the students' responses, to have a record of which questions were answered correctly.

Performance

Performance testing involves hands-on skill and should follow these guidelines:
- Give clear directions of what and how the procedure is to be performed.
- Include a skills check sheet, listing the qualities or standards the educator will be judging. Assign a percentage of the total score for each question. This method will help ensure a more-objective testing session.

Written

Written testing is usually the most objective testing tool. Written test items test the student's recall, recognition, or a combination of both. There are eight types of written questions, which are discussed in chapter 10.

94

10 Constructing Effective Written Tests

Writing an effective written test takes careful planning. It is difficult, perhaps impossible, to construct a perfect test. Even so, the educators' goal is to construct a test that is as fair and objective as possible.

"Garbage-in, garbage-out." This common saying appears to hold true. Most untrained educators compile a list of questions for student testing after a presentation; this is not testing, but a list of random questions. Test questions should directly reflect meeting the stated course objectives. If they do not measure the course objectives, then the educator is wasting both the students' and his or her time and effort.

Test items are basic building blocks and should have only one correct answer. It should be written clearly, so there can be only one interpretation. Professional test-writing services spend many thousands of dollars in writing and rewriting test questions, and some questions are still misunderstood.

Testing Guidelines

The following list is prepared as a guideline in creating written tests:

- Give advanced notice for testing, to allow students adequate time to prepare.
- Provide good test copy; poor test copy is a reflection of the educator as a professional. The test copy should contain correct spelling, grammar, and punctuation, and should be easily readable, not third-generation photocopy. Test should be printed in minimum 12-point, clear font type for constructing tests and double spaces between each question, with adequate space for answers.
- Design test content to measure fundamental knowledge and skills. For example:

  To test students on knowledge associated with the ear as a sensory organ, the test should ask what otitis media is, rather than asking the shape of the incus.

- Design the test format for easy use and easy grading.
- Design the test for the level of understanding of the students. The same test should not be used for registered nurses and nursing assistants.
- Keep wording of the questions simple and direct. Remember that the test is to be designed to test knowledge, not reading ability.
- Construct questions with careful wording so the question cannot be misread or misunderstood. Read over each question after construction, to ensure that it is understandable and cannot be misinterpreted.
- Avoid trick questions; they only reflect who noticed the trick question.

- Design test questions to reinforce learning, not for student failure.
- Tell students before the test that if they have a question or need assistance to raise their hand. If a student did not understand the question, help him or her to understand the question; then, perhaps reword or revise the question for the next test.
- Include written instructions for each type of test and test question, such as these examples:

  "Please place the number in front of the correct answer."

  "Please circle the most correct answer from the four following answers."

Open-book tests are valuable to use for reinforcing book material or to have the students become familiar at locating information. Open-book tests do not test for recall, but reinforce the content material.

Group testing can be done by dividing the class into groups of three, and used effectively in problem-solving testing.

The educator should stay in the room during testing to be available for student questions and, being in the room minimizes opportunities for cheating.

Helpful Hints in Written Test Construction

Constructing a test takes time and effort, so once it is constructed, it should be placed into a test bank, ideally in a computer test bank. Tests should be revised each year, or, in some cases, more frequently to keep information current. Revising a test can be easily accomplished by changing the arrangement of the questions, deleting, or rewriting poorly constructed questions, and by eliminating outdated test questions.

When the same test is to be used frequently, it's good practice to print copies of the test on brightly-colored paper, then insert the tests into a plastic cover sheets. Number each test at the top—#1, #2, etc. Create a separate answer sheet for students to use when completing the test. Ask students to write the corresponding number of the test (i.e., #1, #2, etc.) at the top of the answer sheet in the space provided. This method works well for two primary reasons:

1. Brightly colored paper is easily identifiable and less likely to be shuffled into the student's other papers and then misplaced or lost. If a test is missing after class, the number on the student's answer sheet identifies which student has the test. Tell the class before the test that if all tests are not accounted for, they will automatically receive a failing grade. If a test bank is used, change the arrangement of the questions immediately, if the test cannot be located. It is a good idea to change the arrangement of the test questions at frequent intervals on a regular basis in any case.

2. Encasing tests in plastic protector sheets prevents students from writing on the test sheet. This seems to happen often, even when the test

contains directions written in large letters on the master test that clearly state, "Please place answers on separate answer sheet."

Individual test sheets are easy to grade and easy to store. Make a master copy of the correct questions on a plastic overhead sheet, place it over the test and the incorrect answers are very easy to identify and correct.

Design test questions that are easy to correct; this saves time for the educator. Educators may wish to have the students correct the tests before they leave the classroom. Correcting tests in this way accomplishes two important objectives. If a student inadvertently misses a question, then the student will have the correct information and rationale upon leaving the classroom. Also, this method eliminates the time it takes the educator to correct each individual test.

Create your own post-item analysis after each test is given, to pick up questions that are frequently misinterpreted. All tests should be reviewed, revised, and rewritten at least yearly or as needed. A test analysis can be accomplished easily and quickly, whether using one's own designed evaluation tool (test) or an existing evaluation tool, by following these steps:

1. On blank paper or on the computer, list the question number.

2. Tabulate, opposite the test question number, how many students missed question #1, #2, #3, and so on.

3. If, for example, question # 2 was missed by a
    large number of students in the class, then per-
    haps the question should be rewritten for more
    clarification, or a more thorough explanation
    may need to be given by the educator to the
    students regarding the subject of that question.

Types and Values of Written Test Questions

True/False

True/false questions are the easiest to design and
correct but are the weakest type of test question for
assessing student performance. True/false questions leave a 50-50 chance of guessing the correct
answer. They have been used for testing at the end
of a one-hour in-service because true/false questions can be used to reinforce important facts, such
as, "A nurse is considered negligent if he or she
carries out an order by the physician that is not
safe or correct."

Print the letters "T" and "F" in a column on the
left side of the answer sheet and instruct the student to circle the preprinted letter, to answer the
question; then there can be no mistake as to the
answer. A true/false test is easy to correct:

1. Make a copy of the answer sheet on overhead
    transparency film.

2. Circle the correct answers in dark pen or over-
    head pencil, on the transparency copy of the
    answer sheet.

3. Correct tests by placing the overhead sheet over

each student's test answer sheets, and the incorrect numbers are visible and easy to correct.

Here are examples of true/false formatting, one difficult and one easy:

Difficult format to correct

1. The dominant intracellular electrolyte is sodium. T F

2. Normal saline is considered to be an isotonic solution. T F

Easy format to correct

1. T F   The dominant intracellular electrolyte is sodium.

2. T F   Normal saline is considered to be an isotonic solution.

Matching

Matching questions test the student's abilities in recognition. Make the space for the correct answer at the left margin for easy correction with a master transparency sheet; this format is easy to correct. Place simply worded, short descriptions into the column at the right. Always include an extra short description, so there is one more description than answers. Use no more than 10 items.

Directions to students: Place the correct letter in the space at the left side of the paper. Letters can be used once. Not all the letters will be used.

Here is an example of a matching test:

_____1. urethra   a. tube between the kidney to the bladder

_____2. ureter   b. canal between the bladder and the outside of the body

c. pouch-like protrusion of the urethral wall

Multiple Choice

Multiple choice questions test recognition, recall, and problem solving. Good multiple choice questions are difficult to construct, but effective at measuring the degree of student learning. There should be at least four possible answers. Make at least two or three answers close to the correct answer. Do not make one answer so ridiculous that it is obviously wrong. Multiple choice questions are designed to test recognition and recall based on the learner's prior knowledge and experience, the reason multiple choice questions are used in state board examinations.

Directions to students: Circle the most correct answer from the following four choices.

Here is a *correct* example of a multiple choice test question:

To immobilize a suspected fracture of the tibia, it is best to apply a splint from

a. above the ankle to below the ankle

b. above the knee to below the knee

c. above the knee to below the ankle

d. below the knee to above the ankle

Constructing questions in the correct manner better assures the educator that the student knows the rationale of the procedure, and that immobilization should include the joint both above and below the suspected fracture.

Here is an *incorrect* example of a multiple choice test question:

To immobilize a suspected fracture of the tibia, it is best to apply a splint from

a. above the knee to below the ankle

b. above the knee to below the knee

c. below the waist to above the knee

d. below the nose to the above waist

The selections in the incorrect example are not reflective of a good multiple choice answers. Two of the answers are so unbelievable, it leaves only two real choices, or a 50-50 chance that the student that does not know the rationale but could still select the right answer.

Completion

Completion questions test recall. This type of question is used when a specific technical term, fact, or principle is to be reinforced or remembered. When designing test questions, use only one blank per sentence, and make all answer fill-in lines the same length. Place the space near the end of the sentence, to elicit only the correct answer.

Directions to students: On the blank answer line at the end of the sentence, write in the correct answer.

Example of an incorrect completion question:

_____ is the normal _____
for_____.

Fill-in questions constructed in this way leave much to interpretation and are unclear.

Example of a correct completion question:

The normal oral temperature for an adult is

_____.

The example of this completion question leaves little to misinterpretation and elicits only one correct answer.

Identification

Identification questions test recall and recognition. Identification questions are useful for the student to identify technical parts or objects. This type of question works well when students are unsure how to correctly spell the term. Having the correct spelling and name of the term written on the answer sheet for identification reinforces learning. Asking the student to place the correct letter in the answer space saves time for the student and is easy to correct.

Directions to students: Choose the correct name of the four chambers of the heart from the list that fits the letters on the diagram (diagram would be included).

1. _____ Right atrium

2. _____ Left atrium

3. _____ Left ventricle

4. _____ Right ventricle

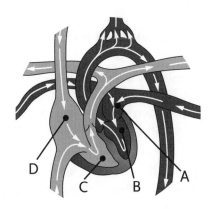

Math

Mathematics and problem-solving questions test both recall and recognition. The educator should make the questions realistic and reflective of common math problems the students will encounter in job situations. This type of question depends upon the level of skill the educator expects the student to demonstrate. Consider this example:

> 1000 cc of D5W is to run 8 hours. Using a 10-drop administration set, how many cc/hr? and/or how many drops per minute?

If the educator wishes to see the students' calculation work on the problem, then the educator should provide the students adequate space to display their calculations.

Directions to students: Answer the following questions, and show calculations on how you arrived at the answer.

Short Answer

Short-answer questions test recall. The short-answer question tends to be more objective. Short-answer questions should be graded on content, not writing ability; therefore, grading may become subjective. Let the students know in advance whether grading criteria will include correct spelling. For students who have difficulty writing English, construct a question that asks the student to circle the answer or answers instead of asking them to write the answers. Constructing short-answer questions in this way makes it easier for the student to complete and easier for the educator to grade.

Here is an example of a short answer test question:

Circle the three common methods of taking a temperature on an eight-month-old pediatric patient.

Axillary

Tympanic

Rectally

Orally

Essay

Essay questions test the student's problem-solving

ability. Essay questions require judgment and are the choice for students who require written, procedural understanding. Students should be given guidelines as to length, time frame, and whether sentence structure, grammar, or spelling will be included as part of the grading criteria. Essay questions are not one of the most effective ways to test skills. Essay questions work well with higher-level students. Essay questions may become subjective in nature because, for example, if an essay is written neatly and contains correct spelling and sentence construction, it appeals to the educator more than the same content that is difficult to read and contains spelling mistakes.

Other Methods for Measuring Student Performance

Skills testing by educator observation

Skills testing is the application of actual generalization or factual data to a problem in clinical demonstration. Conducting skills testing and/or clinical observation makes it more difficult for the educator to be objective. If clinical performance is being tested in the classroom or skills lab, make a checklist of items that each student must perform adequately, and check them off as each student completes each step correctly. Developing a skills checklist keeps the testing fair and objective, and provides the educator with documentation for records.

Products or models

Medical supply and pharmaceutical vendors are eager to provide products for demonstration purposes to medical facilities. The more varieties of visual and hands-on material the educator can provide, the more the learning process is improved for the student.

Projects or posters created by the students

Projects or posters developed either individually or as a group encourage creativity, teamwork, and learning.

11 Making the Grade

Grading is used for purposes of measuring student progress toward stated goals and, also, for use as a motivator for the students. If grades are to be assigned, different types of grading methods may be employed. Grading methods in a vocational school or college are usually established and standardized. If the educator chooses not to assign a number or letter grade and elects to use a pass/fail grading system, the educator needs to establish a standard pass/fail policy and share that policy with the students.

Two common methods of grading are the bell curve and a predetermined percentage of correct answers.

Bell Curve or Normal Distribution Test

This grading method assigns a letter or numeric score, for example, "A" to "F" with "A" being the highest possible grade and "F" the lowest score obtained by the class as a whole. A disadvantage of the bell curve system of grading is that it is not always reflective of true learning and may result in varied grades for the individual depending on the size of the class and knowledge of other students in the class.

If an "A" is given to the student who has the most correct answers and, of that group tested, only one student answered five of ten answers correctly, would it be fair to assign that student an "A"? In retrospect, if only one student succeeded in correctly answering only five questions correct out of ten, then perhaps this may be the time to reevaluate the test questions as well as the teaching methods.

Percentage Grading

Percentage grading is the fairest method of grading. Educators in student learning situations in which grades are required documentation for education programs use the percentage method more often. The passing or acceptable score is usually 70% or 75%. This percentage is predetermined either by the facility, department, nursing board, or the educator. The educator may also choose to make his or her own grading scale.

To use a percent grading system, the total number of test questions are divided by the predetermined passing score. The educator needs to let the students know in advance the passing score.

For example, if the test contains 30 questions and the accepted passing score is 75%, multiply 30 (the total number of questions) by 0.75 (predetermined passing score) to get 23 (the passing number of test questions needed to be answered correctly to obtain a 75% passing score).

To score each test paper, divide the total number of correct questions on the test by the total number of test questions and that will give a percentage grade.

Here is an example:

> Susan answered 26 questions correctly.
> Dividing 26 (correct questions) by 30 (total
> number of questions in test) = 86% (final
> grade).

This method can be used on a smaller test. Look at this example:

> There are ten questions on the test. Multiply: 10
> x 0.70 = 7 (number of correct questions to
> obtain a 70% passing score).

If students are correcting their own tests, instruct them to count the correct answers, rather than counting incorrect answers. This results in a more positive climate in the classroom; counting correct answers is psychologically more motivating than counting incorrect answers.

Name:

In-Service Topic:

Instructor's Name:

Please take a few moments to evaluate the in-service while it is still fresh in your mind. Your honest opinions will help us improve future courses.

For each of the following statements, circle the number that best describes whether you:

1 Strongly Agree
2 Agree
3 Neutral
4 Disagree
5 Strongly Disagree

The instructor was well prepared.
1   2   3   4   5

The instructor knew the subject very well.
1   2   3   4   5

The instructor noticed when I did not understand.
1   2   3   4   5

The correct amount of time was spent on each topic.
1   2   3   4   5

Difficult terms were explained.
1   2   3   4   5

The examples used related to my job.
1   2   3   4   5

I understood the material being presented.
1   2   3   4   5

The visual aids were very good.
1   2   3   4   5

The instructor made learning the material fun.
1   2   3   4   5

The instructor kept the discussion to the topic.
1   2   3   4   5

The instructor kept me interested in the topic.
1   2   3   4   5

My participation in discussions was encouraged.
1   2   3   4   5

Answers to questions were clear.
1   2   3   4   5

The assessment was too hard.
1   2   3   4   5

The assessment was too easy.
1   2   3   4   5

The handouts were easy to understand.
1   2   3   4   5

The handouts were helpful.
1   2   3   4   5

Overall, this in-service was very good.
1   2   3   4   5

Additional comments:

12 Constructing Evaluations

The evaluation form is another important measurement tool used in teaching. The evaluation form gathers feedback information about the learner's opinion of the course. Post-course evaluations provide information on how the student perceived the course in terms of meeting individual needs and how the student perceived the educator's mastery of the subject.

The student course evaluation should be designed to gather pertinent information that will assist the educator in determining whether the content, conditions, and goals of the class were perceived as being met by the students. Evaluations can be an invaluable feedback tool for use in revising and improving the course.

Five suggested aspects that may be measured are as follows:

1. Extent to which the course met the objectives

2. Instructor's knowledge of the subject

3. Use of appropriate teaching methods

4. Usefulness of the new information

5. Other areas the educator wants as specific information

The educator may wish to ask, "Please list other class topics you would like presented that would be of benefit to you." This question elicits a response from students to list course suggestions that would benefit them, rather than asking, "What would you like presented?"

The educator should use questions that are relevant. In a large facility where other educators will be presenting courses, the staff director may wish to evaluate the attitude of the individual educators. What better way than by feedback from students? Questions that directly evaluate the educators might be asked, such as these:

> Did the instructor start class on time?

> Did the instructor involve all students in discussions and presentations?

Ideally, evaluations should be used at the end of each course, but for short, thirty-minute or one-hour in-service presentations, the nurse educator may do evaluations monthly or at scheduled intervals. Gathering up evaluations and immediately placing them into a storage file is a useless exercise; evaluations should be read and used as the valuable feedback tool for which they were intended.

Use evaluations to revise and improve the course. A competent educator can gather useful information from the evaluations by reading between the lines. Evaluations that consistently have negative comments or no comments at all may stem from the overall attitude of the instructor. A competent and creative educator can conduct a class in a rain-storm and get positive evaluations, while a poor educator can present a class under the most ideal conditions and receive negative evaluations.